The Comprehensive Guide to Dog Grooming : Keeping Your Dog Happy and Healthy

Melissa Groomer

No part of this book may be reproduced, stored in a retrieval system, or transmitted in any form or by any means, electronic, mechanical, photocopying, recording, or otherwise, without prior written permission from the publisher.

DEDICATION

To the loyal companions who fill our lives with boundless joy and unwavering companionship. This book is dedicated to every dog lover, groomer, and caregiver who embraces the art and science of nurturing our beloved furry friends. May these pages serve as a compass, guiding you through the grooming journey, fostering a deeper bond and enhancing the well-being of our cherished canine companions.

CONTENT

ACKNOWLEDGMENTS

I extend my heartfelt gratitude to the countless dogs whose presence and personalities have been a constant source of inspiration. Their patience during grooming sessions and their unconditional love from the core of this book.

I am deeply indebted to the expert groomers, veterinarians, and professionals in the field whose knowledge, guidance, and valuable insights have shaped this comprehensive guide.

Special thanks to my family and friends for their unwavering support, understanding, and encouragement throughout the creation of this book. Your love and understanding of my passion for dogs have been instrumental in bringing this project to life.

I also express my appreciation to the publishers, editors, designers, and everyone involved in the production of this book. Your dedication and hard work have transformed this vision into a reality.

Lastly, to all the dog enthusiasts and readers embarking on this grooming journey, I thank you. Your commitment to the well-being and happiness of our four-legged companions is both commendable and inspiring. May this guide contribute to the health and joy of the dogs in your life.

Chapter 1: Understanding Your Dog's Coat and Grooming Needs

1. **Introduction to Coat Types:**

- Short, Medium, Long, Double-Coated, and Wire-Haired Breeds: Define and explain different coat types found in dogs.

- Characteristics of Each Coat Type: Highlight the specific attributes, shedding tendencies, and grooming needs associated with each type.

2. **Assessing Your Dog's Coat:**

- Determining Coat Type: Describe methods to identify your dog's coat type through visual inspection and tactile examination.

- Special Considerations: Highlight how a dog's age, health, and activities can influence their coat condition and grooming needs.

3. **Grooming Needs Based on Coat Type:**

- Short-Haired Breeds: Discuss low-maintenance grooming needs and the significance of regular brushing and bathing.

- Long-Haired Breeds: Explore the necessity for frequent grooming, detangling, and professional grooming assistance.

- Double-Coated and Wire-Haired Breeds: Emphasize the unique requirements, such as deshedding techniques and specific grooming tools.

4. **Tailoring Grooming Routines:**

- Customizing Grooming Regimens: How to adapt grooming schedules and techniques to suit your dog's specific coat type and individual needs.

- Establishing a Routine: Importance of consistency in grooming to maintain a healthy coat and ensure your dog's comfort.

5. **Coat Health and Hygiene:**

- Impact on Overall Health: Discuss how grooming practices contribute to a dog's well-being, preventing skin issues and maintaining hygiene.

- Signs of Coat-Related Problems: Highlight indications of potential health issues visible in the coat.

Conclusion:

- Emphasizing the Role of Understanding Coat Types: Summarize the importance of recognizing and comprehending your dog's coat type to tailor an effective grooming routine for a happy and healthy companion.

This chapter aims to provide a comprehensive understanding of different coat types in dogs, their grooming requirements, and the importance of recognizing individual needs to establish an effective grooming routine.

Chapter 2: Establishing a Grooming Routine

Grooming your dog is not just about aesthetics; it's a vital aspect of their overall health and well-being. Creating a consistent grooming routine is crucial in maintaining their hygiene, preventing health issues, and fostering a strong bond between you and your pet.

Understanding Your Dog's Grooming Needs:

1. **Assessing Coat Type and Breed:** Different breeds have varied grooming requirements. Understand the specifics of your dog's coat type—whether it's short, long, double-coated, curly, or wire-haired—and research the particular needs associated with it.

2. **Frequency of Grooming:** Establish how often your dog needs grooming based on their coat type, lifestyle, and activities. Dogs that spend more time outdoors might require more frequent grooming.

Elements of a Grooming Routine:

1. **Brushing:** Regular brushing removes loose hair, prevents matting, and distributes natural oils in the coat. Determine the appropriate brush type for your dog's coat and establish a consistent brushing schedule.

2. **Bathing:** The frequency of baths depends on your dog's lifestyle and coat. Use dog-specific shampoos and thoroughly rinse to prevent skin irritation. Establish a bathing routine suitable for your dog.

3. **Nail Care:** Trim your dog's nails regularly to prevent overgrowth, discomfort, or potential injury. Acquaint your dog with the tools and process gradually to make it a stress-free experience.

4. **Ear and Eye Care:** Regularly clean your dog's ears and eyes to prevent infections. Use gentle, vet-approved solutions and techniques to maintain cleanliness without causing discomfort.

Creating a Positive Grooming Environment:

1. **Positive Association:** Associate grooming with positive experiences by using treats, praise, and play. This builds a positive connection and reduces anxiety or resistance.

2. **Consistent Environment:** Choose a calm, well-lit area for grooming. Ensure the space is comfortable and free from distractions to help your dog relax during grooming sessions.

Adapting the Routine to Your Dog's Needs:

1. **Observation and Adjustment:** Watch for any signs of discomfort or stress during grooming. Modify the routine as needed to accommodate your dog's comfort level.

2. **Professional Assistance:** Seek guidance from professional groomers or veterinarians, especially if you encounter challenges or are uncertain about specific grooming techniques.

Conclusion:

Establishing a grooming routine involves patience, consistency, and attentiveness. By understanding your dog's needs and preferences, and creating a positive grooming environment, you'll not only maintain their physical health but also strengthen the bond between you and your furry companion.

Chapter 3: Brushing and Bathing

- ☐ Understanding the right brushing techniques for different coat types
- ☐ Proper bathing techniques, frequency, and using appropriate shampoos,
- ☐ Drying methods and tools for different coats.

Brushing and bathing are fundamental components of a dog's grooming routine. These activities not only maintain your dog's appearance but also contribute significantly to their overall health and well-being.

Brushing Your Dog:

1. **Understanding Coat Types:** Different coat types require specific brushing techniques and tools. Determine whether your dog has a short, long, double, curly, or wire-haired coat and select appropriate brushes or combs.

2. **Regular Brushing Schedule:** Establish a consistent brushing routine. Some dogs may need daily brushing to prevent matting and remove loose hair, while others might require brushing every few days.

3. **Proper Technique:** Brush in the direction of hair growth, starting from the head and moving towards the tail. Be gentle, especially around sensitive areas, and untangle any mats gradually to avoid discomfort.

4. **Addressing Specific Needs:** Pay attention to areas that are prone to matting, such as behind the ears, underarms, and the belly. Use detangling spray if needed, and be patient when dealing with knots.

Bathing Your Dog:

1. **Determining Bath Frequency:** Decide on a bathing schedule based on your dog's activity level and coat type. Some dogs may require baths every few weeks, while others might need them less frequently to avoid stripping the coat of natural oils.

2. **Choosing the Right Shampoo:** Use dog-specific shampoos that suit your dog's skin type. Avoid using human shampoos as they can cause skin irritation due to differences in pH levels.

3. **Preparing for the Bath:** Brush your dog before bathing to remove loose hair and prevent tangling. Place a non-slip mat in the bathtub to ensure your dog feels secure.

4. **Bathing Technique:** Use lukewarm water and wet your dog thoroughly, avoiding water in the ears and eyes. Gently massage shampoo into the coat, starting from the neck and working towards the tail. Rinse the shampoo completely to prevent skin irritation.

5. **Drying Your Dog:** Use towels to remove excess water and avoid vigorous rubbing. If your dog is comfortable, use a blow dryer on a low, warm setting. Be cautious around sensitive areas and keep the dryer at a safe distance to prevent burns.

Adapting to Your Dog's Preferences:

- Monitor your dog's reaction during brushing and bathing. If they seem anxious or uncomfortable, adjust the process and provide positive reinforcement to create a pleasant experience.

Conclusion:

Regular brushing and bathing are essential for your dog's health and appearance. By understanding your dog's coat type, using the right tools and techniques, and being mindful of their comfort, you can ensure that grooming sessions become a positive and beneficial experience for both you and your furry friend.

Chapter 4: Nail Trimming and Paw Care

Nail trimming guidelines and tools
Caring for paw pads and between toes
Handling and calming dogs during paw maintenance

Proper nail trimming and paw care are essential aspects of
your dog's grooming routine. Neglecting these areas can

lead to discomfort, pain, and potential health issues. Understanding the techniques and tools necessary for nail care and paw maintenance is crucial for your dog's overall well-being.

Nail Trimming:

1. **Understanding Nail Anatomy:** Get familiar with your dog's nails and the quick—the blood vessel and nerves inside the nail. Cutting into the quick can cause bleeding and pain.

2. **Tools for Nail Trimming:** Invest in high-quality nail clippers specifically designed for dogs. You may also use a nail grinder for smoother edges. Have styptic powder on hand in case of accidental bleeding.

3. **Getting Your Dog Accustomed:** Introduce your dog to the nail trimming tools gradually. Let them sniff and inspect the clippers or grinder without any pressure. This helps reduce anxiety.

4. **Proper Trimming Technique:** Trim a small bit of the nail at a time, staying clear of the quick. Focus on visible white or clear parts of the nail and avoid the pink area, which indicates the presence of the quick.

5. **Reassurance and Reward:** If your dog is anxious, provide reassurance and rewards during and after the trimming process. Ensure the experience is positive to build trust and reduce stress.

Paw Care:

1. **Inspecting Paws Regularly:** Check your dog's paws for any signs of injury, foreign objects, or overgrown hair. Clean gently if necessary and monitor for redness or swelling.

2. **Trimming Paw Hair:** Some dogs, especially those with long hair, may require trimming around the paw pads to prevent matting and debris collection. Use blunt-end scissors and be cautious to avoid accidentally cutting the skin.

3. **Moisturizing Paw Pads:** Use dog-safe moisturizers or paw balms to keep paw pads hydrated, especially in extreme weather conditions.

4. **Protective Measures:** Consider using dog booties or protective paw waxes in challenging environments, such as extreme heat, cold, or rough terrains, to prevent injuries and damage to the paws.

Adapting to Your Dog's Needs:

- Observe your dog's reaction during nail trimming and paw care. If they show signs of discomfort or anxiety, adjust your approach and introduce the activities gradually.

Conclusion:

Regular nail trimming and paw care are essential for your dog's comfort and mobility. By employing the right tools, techniques, and gradual introduction to these grooming activities, you ensure a positive experience and maintain your dog's paws in healthy condition, contributing to their overall well-being.

Chapter 5: Ear and Eye Care

- ☐ Safely cleaning ears and managing ear hair
- ☐ Gentle eye cleaning methods
- ☐ Recognizing signs of infection or discomfort

Ear and eye care are crucial components of your dog's grooming routine. Proper maintenance of these areas not only ensures your dog's comfort but also contributes to their overall health and well-being. Understanding the correct techniques and tools for ear and eye care is essential to prevent infections and maintain your dog's sensory health.

Ear Care:

1. **Regular Inspection:** Regularly examine your dog's ears for signs of redness, swelling, unusual odor, or discharge. Any such indications may signal an infection or ear issues.

2. **Cleaning Process:** Use a vet-recommended ear cleaning solution and soft cotton balls or pads to gently wipe the visible part of the ear canal. Avoid inserting anything deep into the ear canal as it may cause damage.

3. **Ear Hair Management:** Some breeds grow hair inside the ear canal, which can lead to wax buildup or infections. Trim this hair carefully to maintain cleanliness but be cautious not to cause any injuries.

4. **Professional Check-ups:** If you notice any abnormalities in your dog's ears or if they show signs of discomfort, consult your vet for a thorough examination.

Eye Care:

1. **Regular Eye Inspection:** Check your dog's eyes for any discharge, redness, cloudiness, or signs of irritation. If you notice any abnormalities, seek veterinary advice promptly.

2. **Cleaning Technique:** Use a vet-approved eye cleaning solution or a damp, clean cloth to gently wipe around the eye area. Be cautious not to touch the eyeball directly.

3. **Tear Stain Management:** Some dogs may develop tear stains, especially around light-colored fur. Use tear stain removers or consult your vet for safe and effective solutions to manage this issue.

4. **Seeking Professional Help:** If your dog shows persistent signs of eye discomfort, excessive tearing, or squinting, it's crucial to seek prompt veterinary attention.

Adapting to Your Dog's Needs:

- Introduce ear and eye care gradually, offering treats and praise to ensure a positive association. If your dog seems uncomfortable, adjust the process and seek professional guidance if necessary.

Conclusion:

Regular ear and eye care are vital for your dog's sensory health. By employing gentle cleaning techniques, regular inspection, and seeking professional help when needed, you can ensure your dog's comfort and prevent potential health issues, contributing significantly to their overall well-being.

Chapter 6: Grooming Specific Breeds

- [ ] Breed-specific grooming requirements and techniques
- [ ] Show grooming vs. practical, everyday grooming for different breeds

Each dog breed has unique characteristics and grooming requirements. Understanding the distinct needs of different breeds is vital for ensuring their coats, skin, and overall health are properly maintained. Tailoring your grooming routine to suit the specific demands of your dog's breed will help keep them healthy and looking their best.

Short-Haired Breeds:

1. **Grooming Needs:** Breeds like Beagles, Boxers, and Dalmatians have short, smooth coats that require minimal grooming. Regular brushing to remove loose hair and occasional baths suffice for these breeds.

2. **Care Emphasis:** Focus on nail trimming, ear cleaning, and dental care. Short-haired breeds may require less attention to coat grooming but still need overall hygiene maintenance.

Long-Haired Breeds:

1. **Grooming Needs:** Breeds like Shih Tzus, Maltese, and Afghan Hounds have long, flowing coats that demand extensive grooming. Regular brushing and detangling to prevent mats and knots are essential.
2. **Care Emphasis:** Use specific brushes and combs suitable for long hair to maintain their coat. Pay close attention to areas prone to matting, such as behind the ears and under the legs.

Double-Coated Breeds:

1. **Grooming Needs:** Breeds like German Shepherds, Huskies, and Golden Retrievers have a dense undercoat beneath their topcoat. They shed heavily, especially during shedding seasons, and require consistent brushing to manage shedding.
2. **Care Emphasis:** Invest in quality deshedding tools to remove loose undercoat fur and prevent mats. Be cautious not to damage the undercoat while grooming.

Curly-Coated Breeds:

1. **Grooming Needs:** Breeds like Poodles, Bichon Frises, and Portuguese Water Dogs have curly, non-shedding coats that require regular grooming to prevent matting and tangles.
2. **Care Emphasis:** Regular brushing and professional grooming every 4-6 weeks are essential for

curly-coated breeds. Trimming to maintain the desired shape is also important.

Wire-Haired Breeds:

1. **Grooming Needs:** Breeds like Wire Fox Terriers, Schnauzers, and Dachshunds have coarse, wiry coats that require specific attention to maintain their unique texture.
2. **Care Emphasis:** Regular brushing and hand-stripping are necessary for wire-haired breeds to manage shedding and maintain the coat's texture. Trimming might also be required to keep a neat appearance.

Specialty Breeds:

1. **Grooming Needs:** Breeds such as the Komondor or the Bedlington Terrier have unique coats that require specific grooming techniques to maintain their characteristic appearance.
2. **Care Emphasis:** Seek professional advice or specialized grooming techniques tailored to these breeds' distinctive coats to maintain their individual traits and textures.

Adapting to Breed-Specific Requirements:

- Understand the unique grooming needs of your dog's breed. Tailor your grooming routine and tools to suit those requirements to ensure the best care and appearance for your furry friend.

Conclusion:

Each breed has distinct grooming needs. By understanding and accommodating these specific requirements in your grooming routine, you can maintain your dog's coat, skin, and overall health effectively while ensuring they look their best according to their breed's unique characteristics.

Chapter 7: Tricky Areas: Face, Tail, and Anal Glands

- [ ] Delicate grooming techniques for sensitive areas
- [ ] Managing facial hair, tail hygiene, and anal gland care

Certain areas of a dog's body require delicate grooming and attention to maintain hygiene and prevent potential health issues. Addressing the face, tail, and anal glands appropriately is essential in ensuring your dog's overall comfort and well-being.

Face Grooming:

1. **Sensitive Care:** The face is a delicate area that requires gentle grooming. Use soft brushes or grooming wipes to clean around the eyes, muzzle, and folds on breeds with wrinkled faces.

2. **Eye and Tear Stain Maintenance:** Some breeds are prone to tear stains. Use vet-approved products or

remedies to manage and prevent tear stains without causing irritation.

3. **Hair Trimming:** Trim hair around the eyes carefully to prevent obstruction of vision. Use blunt-end scissors or seek professional help for breeds with hair that grows close to their eyes.

Tail Hygiene:

1. **Regular Inspection:** Check your dog's tail for any signs of injury, skin issues, or foreign objects that might cause discomfort.

2. **Brushing and Detangling:** For breeds with long tail fur, brush and detangle carefully to prevent matting and remove debris.

3. **Trimming:** Some dogs might need tail hair trimmed to maintain cleanliness and prevent tangling. Ensure safe trimming practices to avoid accidents.

Anal Gland Care:

1. **Understanding Anal Glands:** Dogs have anal glands that sometimes need manual expression or may naturally empty during bowel movements. However, issues like impaction or infections can arise, leading to discomfort and health problems.

2. **Symptom Recognition:** Watch for signs of anal gland problems, such as scooting, licking, or foul odor. If you notice these signs, consult a veterinarian promptly.

3. **Professional Help:** If your dog's anal glands require expression, it's advisable to seek help from a professional groomer or veterinarian experienced in this procedure.

Adapting to Your Dog's Comfort:

- Introduce grooming in these sensitive areas gradually and positively. Use treats and praise to ensure a comfortable and stress-free experience for your dog.

Conclusion:

Grooming the face, tail, and addressing anal gland care necessitates a gentle and cautious approach. By maintaining these areas with care and addressing any specific issues promptly, you ensure your dog's comfort and reduce the risk of potential health problems, contributing to their overall well-being.

Chapter 8: Grooming for Health and Wellness

- ☐ How grooming contributes to a dog's overall health
- ☐ Detecting skin issues, parasites, or abnormalities during grooming

Grooming goes beyond aesthetics; it significantly impacts a dog's health and overall well-being. Understanding how grooming practices contribute to a dog's physical health, emotional state, and comfort is vital for responsible pet care.

Skin and Coat Health:

1. **Regular Brushing and Bathing:** Routine brushing eliminates dead hair, distributes natural oils, and prevents matting. Regular baths with appropriate shampoos maintain skin health, removing dirt and preventing skin issues.

2. **Detection of Skin Issues:** During grooming, closely inspect your dog's skin for abnormalities, lumps, ticks, fleas, or signs of infection. Early detection aids in prompt treatment.

3. **Coat-Specific Care:** Tailor grooming techniques to suit your dog's coat type to maintain its health. For example, proper grooming for double-coated breeds assists in the shedding process, preventing mats and ensuring air circulation.

Dental and Ear Health:

1. **Teeth Cleaning:** Regularly brushing your dog's teeth and providing dental treats or toys contributes to oral health, preventing plaque and tartar buildup.

2. **Ear Care:** Gently clean ears to prevent wax buildup, infections, or mites. Regular maintenance ensures your dog's ear health and prevents potential issues.

Preventing Parasites:

1. **Flea and Tick Prevention:** Grooming provides the opportunity to check for and remove ticks and fleas. Use preventive treatments recommended by your veterinarian to protect your dog from parasites.

2. **Worm Control:** Regular grooming sessions allow for early detection of signs of worms or other parasites. Follow your vet's advice on deworming and preventive measures.

Emotional Well-being:

1. **Bonding and Trust:** Grooming sessions are valuable bonding moments. Positive interaction during grooming builds trust and strengthens the bond between you and your dog.

2. **Stress Reduction:** Regular grooming in a calm, positive environment reduces stress for your dog. Consistency and positive reinforcement create a relaxed grooming experience.

Monitoring Overall Health:

1. **Physical Condition Observation:** Grooming sessions offer the chance to observe your dog's physical condition. Changes in weight, lumps, or abnormalities can be detected early.

2. **Comfort and Mobility:** Keeping nails trimmed and paws well-maintained ensures your dog's comfort and proper mobility.

Conclusion:

Grooming is an integral part of maintaining a dog's health and wellness. Regular grooming not only ensures your dog looks and smells good but also plays a crucial role in their physical health, emotional state, and the bond between you and your furry companion. It is a holistic approach that supports your dog's overall well-being.

Chapter 9: Troubleshooting Common Grooming Challenges

- ☐ Addressing matting, tangles, and excessive shedding
- ☐ Handling nervous or uncooperative dogs during grooming

Grooming can present various challenges, from matting to a dog's resistance during nail trimming or bathing. Understanding and addressing these common issues are essential for maintaining a positive grooming experience for both you and your furry friend.

Matting and Tangles:

1. **Prevention:** Regular brushing and appropriate grooming tools can prevent mats and tangles. Begin with detangling spray or conditioner for easier removal.

2. **Untangling Technique:** Gently separate the mat with your fingers and use a wide-tooth comb or slicker brush. Work from the outside of the mat towards the center to avoid causing discomfort.

Resistance to Nail Trimming:

1. **Gradual Introduction:** Start by getting your dog accustomed to the sight and sound of nail clippers without any pressure. Offer treats and positive reinforcement to create a positive association.

2. **Slow Progress:** Gradually move from introducing the clippers to gently touching the paws. Reward your dog for allowing the handling.

Bathing Challenges:

1. **Comfortable Environment:** Ensure a calm, non-slippery bathing area and introduce your dog to the process gradually.

2. **Positive Reinforcement:** Use treats, praise, and patience during baths to create a positive experience.

Ear and Eye Sensitivity:

1. **Gentle Approach:** Use vet-approved solutions and soft materials for sensitive areas. Avoid direct contact with the eyes and gently clean around them.

2. **Positive Reinforcement:** Reward your dog during and after ear and eye care to associate the experience with positivity.

Excessive Shedding:

1. **Regular Brushing:** Implement a consistent brushing routine to remove loose hair and prevent shedding.

2. **Proper Nutrition:** Ensure your dog's diet contains essential nutrients that promote a healthy coat.

Managing Anxiety and Stress:

1. **Calm Environment:** Choose a quiet, well-lit space for grooming and eliminate potential stress triggers.

2. **Gradual Exposure:** Introduce grooming activities slowly and positively to reduce anxiety.

Handling Uncooperative Behavior:

1. **Patience and Consistency:** Stay calm and patient during grooming sessions. Pause and resume grooming if your dog becomes too stressed.

2. **Professional Help:** If you encounter persistent challenges, seek guidance from professional groomers or trainers for tips on handling resistant behavior.

Conclusion:

Encountering challenges during grooming is common, but with patience, gradual introduction, and positive reinforcement, many issues can be managed effectively. Understanding your dog's behavior and employing appropriate techniques will help overcome these challenges

and create a more comfortable grooming experience for
your furry companion.

Chapter 10: Professional Grooming vs. DIY Grooming

- ☐ Pros and cons of professional grooming services
- ☐ Tips for grooming at home and when to seek professional help

The choice between professional grooming and grooming your dog at home involves various considerations, each with its advantages and potential drawbacks. Understanding the differences between the two options can help you make an informed decision that best suits your dog's needs and your preferences.

Professional Grooming:

Advantages:

1. **Expertise and Skill:** Professional groomers are trained and experienced in various grooming

techniques, especially for specific breeds and coat types.

2. **Specialized Equipment:** They have access to professional-grade tools and products, ensuring an efficient and thorough grooming process.

3. **Comprehensive Services:** Services often include nail trimming, ear cleaning, anal gland expression, and specific breed trims, which might be challenging for amateurs.

4. **Time-Saving:** Professional groomers can provide a quicker and more efficient grooming experience.

Considerations:

1. **Cost:** Professional grooming services can be more expensive compared to DIY grooming sessions.

2. **Scheduling:** Availability and appointments may not always align with your preferred times, leading to potential inconvenience.

3. **Stress Reduction:** Some dogs might feel more relaxed and less anxious in a professional grooming environment due to the groomer's expertise and the salon atmosphere.

DIY Grooming:

Advantages:

1. **Cost-Efficiency:** Grooming at home can be more cost-effective in the long run, especially if you invest in quality tools.

2. **Bonding Experience:** Grooming your dog at home fosters a strong bond and trust between you and your pet.

3. **Flexibility:** You have the freedom to groom your dog at your convenience without adhering to specific appointment times.

4. **Consistency:** Regular DIY grooming sessions provide consistency, allowing you to track changes in your dog's health and behavior more closely.

Considerations:

1. **Skill and Knowledge:** DIY grooming requires learning proper techniques and tools suitable for your dog's breed and coat type.

2. **Time and Effort:** Grooming at home might take longer, especially if you're new to the process, and might require more effort to ensure a thorough job.

3. **Potential Stress:** Some dogs might feel anxious or stressed during DIY grooming, especially if they are not used to the process.

Conclusion:

The decision between professional grooming and DIY grooming depends on various factors, including your dog's specific needs, your comfort level with grooming techniques, time availability, and budget. Assessing these considerations will help you determine the best approach that ensures your dog's grooming needs are met effectively and comfortably. It's also possible to combine both methods by utilizing professional services periodically while maintaining grooming practices at home to ensure a well-rounded grooming experience for your furry companion.

Chapter 11: Advanced Grooming Techniques and Creative Styling

- ☐ Advanced grooming skills and tools
- ☐ Exploring creative styling options and popular trends

Beyond the basics of grooming, some advanced techniques and creative styling methods can transform your dog's appearance, showcasing intricate styles and enhancing their overall grooming experience. These advanced techniques require skill, practice, and knowledge of specific breed standards.

Advanced Techniques:

1. **Scissoring and Blending:** Skilled scissoring techniques involve shaping and blending the coat for a neat and balanced look. This method is commonly

used for breeds with specific grooming standards like Poodles or Bichon Frises.

2. **Hand Stripping:** Certain wire-coated breeds require hand-stripping to maintain their coat texture. This process involves pulling out the dead hair manually to encourage new growth.

3. **Creative Coloring:** Non-toxic and pet-safe dyes can be used for creative coloring. This technique adds flair and uniqueness to your dog's appearance, allowing for vibrant or artistic designs.

4. **Asian Fusion Grooming:** A trend that combines traditional grooming with creative and stylish cuts. This method involves sculpting the coat into various shapes and designs.

Breed-Specific Styling:

1. **Show-Cut Styling:** Certain breeds have specific grooming standards for dog shows. Professional groomers are trained in achieving these specific styles according to breed standards.

2. **Asian Style Grooming:** This trend often involves stylized, unique trims and cuts, resulting in creative and eye-catching appearances. It often includes fluffing and shaping the coat to give a teddy bear-like appearance.

Artistic Grooming:

1. **Pom-Pom Styles:** Creating pom-poms on certain areas of the coat, such as the hips or tail, for a unique and playful appearance.

2. **Feathering and Trimming:** Detailed feathering and creative trimming around the ears or paws can enhance the dog's aesthetics.

Safety and Considerations:

1. **Professional Training:** Advanced grooming techniques often require specialized training and practice. Seek guidance from experienced groomers or enroll in grooming courses.

2. **Skin and Coat Health:** Ensure the grooming process does not compromise your dog's skin or coat health. Using quality products and techniques that prioritize your dog's well-being is crucial.

Conclusion:

Advanced grooming techniques and creative styling offer opportunities to showcase your dog's individuality and style. However, these techniques require skill, practice, and attention to your dog's well-being. It's important to understand the breed standards and potential impact on your dog's health before attempting these advanced grooming methods. Professional advice and training can help you achieve these stylish and creative looks while maintaining your dog's health and comfort.

Chapter 12: Grooming Etiquette and Safety

☐ Safety precautions during grooming sessions
☐ Understanding dog behavior and body language during grooming

Maintaining grooming etiquette and ensuring safety measures during grooming sessions are essential for a positive and secure experience for both you and your furry companion. Understanding proper protocols and safety considerations will help create a comfortable and risk-free grooming environment.

Safety Precautions:

1. **Proper Equipment Use:** Ensure grooming tools are in good condition and used correctly to prevent accidents or injuries.

2. **Careful Handling:** Handle your dog gently and patiently during grooming to avoid causing stress or physical discomfort.

3. **Avoidance of Sensitive Areas:** Be cautious around sensitive areas such as eyes, ears, and paws to prevent accidental injuries.

4. **Correct Techniques:** Learn and apply proper grooming techniques to avoid skin irritations or accidental cuts.

5. **Safe Environment:** Use a secure and stable grooming area to prevent slips or falls during the grooming process.

Grooming Etiquette:

1. **Consistency:** Maintain a consistent grooming routine to help your dog become familiar and comfortable with the process.

2. **Positive Reinforcement:** Use treats, praise, and rewards to create a positive association with grooming, encouraging good behavior.

3. **Respectful Approach:** Respect your dog's boundaries and signals. If your dog seems uncomfortable, take a break or adjust the grooming process.

4. **Regular Breaks:** Allow breaks during grooming sessions, especially for longer procedures, to prevent stress or fatigue for your dog.

5. **Cleanliness and Hygiene:** Ensure grooming tools are clean and sanitized to avoid potential infections or skin issues.

Understanding Body Language:

1. **Communication:** Learn to interpret your dog's body language. Signs of discomfort, stress, or resistance should be observed and addressed appropriately.

2. **Handling Stress:** If your dog displays signs of stress or discomfort, such as panting, pacing, or yawning, consider modifying the grooming process or taking a break.

Professional Assistance:

1. **Consultation:** Seek guidance from professional groomers or veterinarians for advice on grooming techniques, especially for advanced procedures.

2. **Professional Services:** If certain grooming tasks seem challenging or stressful for you or your dog, consider seeking professional grooming services.

Conclusion:

Maintaining grooming etiquette and ensuring safety protocols are crucial for a positive grooming experience. Respecting your dog's comfort, employing proper techniques, and being attentive to their body language will help create a secure and pleasant grooming environment. Incorporating positive reinforcement and a respectful approach will not only ensure safety but also strengthen the

bond between you and your beloved pet during grooming
sessions.

41

Chapter 13: The Bond Between Grooming and Dog-Owner Relationship

- Strengthening the bond through grooming
- Using grooming as a form of positive interaction and trust-building

Grooming is far more than a routine task; it plays a significant role in the relationship between a dog and their owner. It's a time for bonding, trust-building, and mutual care. The grooming process enhances the emotional connection and fosters a deeper relationship between you and your furry companion.

Building Trust and Connection:

1. **Establishing Routine:** Through consistent grooming sessions, a sense of predictability and

security is created, fostering trust between you and your dog.

2. **Positive Reinforcement:** Rewarding good behavior during grooming with treats, praise, and affection reinforces the bond and encourages a positive association with the process.

Communication and Understanding:

1. **Body Language Observation:** Grooming provides a valuable opportunity to understand your dog's body language and signals. Recognizing their comfort levels and boundaries strengthens your connection.

2. **Mutual Understanding:** Over time, you'll learn your dog's preferences, dislikes, and individual needs, enhancing your ability to cater to their comfort.

Strengthening the Relationship:

1. **Shared Experience:** Grooming isn't just a task; it's an experience shared between you and your dog, promoting closeness and companionship.

2. **Emotional Bonding:** The physical touch and one-on-one interaction during grooming nurture a special emotional bond between you and your dog.

Care and Wellness:

1. **Health Awareness:** Regular grooming allows for the early detection of health issues, promoting

proactive care and attentiveness to your dog's well-being.

2. **Mutual Care:** Grooming is an act of care and attention from you towards your dog, reinforcing their sense of being loved and cared for.

Grooming as Quality Time:

1. **Relaxation and Comfort:** A calm, quiet grooming environment creates a relaxing atmosphere, promoting a sense of security and comfort for your dog.

2. **Uninterrupted Connection:** Grooming provides undivided attention, allowing for uninterrupted bonding time that enhances the relationship.

Conclusion:

Grooming is more than a grooming session; it's an integral part of the relationship you share with your dog. The time spent grooming is an opportunity for building trust, understanding, and emotional closeness. By approaching grooming as a shared experience and a gesture of care, you're not only maintaining your dog's hygiene but also nurturing a strong, loving, and unbreakable bond between you and your beloved pet.

Chapter 14: Resources and Further Learning

Additional resources, websites, and books for continued learning are very important as well.

Below is a curated list of resources and avenues for further learning and exploration in the realm of dog grooming:

Websites and Online Platforms:

1. **American Kennel Club (AKC):** The AKC website provides breed-specific grooming tips, health guides, and educational resources.

2. **PetMD:** Offers articles, guides, and tips on dog grooming, health, and wellness.

3. **Groomer to Groomer:** A professional grooming industry magazine that shares insights, techniques, and industry trends.

Books:

1. **"Notes from the Grooming Table" by Melissa Verplank:** A comprehensive guide covering grooming techniques and breed-specific styles.

2. **"The Stone Guide to Dog Grooming for All Breeds" by Ben Stone:** A detailed book on grooming techniques for various dog breeds.

Online Courses and Workshops:

1. **The National Dog Groomers Association of America (NDGAA):** Offers certification programs, workshops, and online courses for grooming professionals and enthusiasts.

2. **Udemy:** Provides various online grooming courses suitable for beginners and those looking to advance their grooming skills.

YouTube Channels and Videos:

1. **Sue Zecco:** A professional groomer sharing grooming tutorials, tips, and techniques for various breeds.

2. **The Online Dog Trainer:** Offers grooming videos and insights into dog behavior and training.

Local Grooming Workshops and Seminars:

Look for local grooming workshops, seminars, or events organized by pet stores, grooming salons, or professional associations. These in-person sessions often provide hands-on experience and networking opportunities with experienced groomers.

Local Pet Groomers and Veterinarians:

Establish a relationship with local groomers or veterinarians. They can provide personalized advice, grooming tips, and guidance specific to your dog's needs.

Exploring these resources will offer a wealth of information, guidance, and practical tips to enhance your dog grooming skills and knowledge. Whether you're a beginner or looking to advance your grooming techniques, these avenues provide valuable insights and education for grooming and caring for your furry companion.

Conclusion

This comprehensive guide would cover various aspects of grooming, considering the needs of different dog breeds and their specific coat types. Each chapter could delve into the details and intricacies of maintaining a dog's hygiene and appearance while ensuring their comfort and well-being.

Grooming your dog is an act of care, an opportunity for bonding, and a means of maintaining their health and well-being. It's more than just ensuring your dog looks good; it's about nurturing a strong, loving relationship. By understanding grooming techniques, embracing safety measures, and appreciating the emotional connection it fosters, you create a comfortable and trusting environment for your furry friend.

Remember, grooming is a shared experience that strengthens the bond between you and your dog. It's a journey of learning and growing together, enriching your connection and enhancing the quality of life for your beloved pet. Whether you seek professional assistance or embark on DIY grooming, the key is to approach grooming with patience, love, and a willingness to understand your dog's needs.

In this guide, we've covered grooming basics, advanced techniques, safety measures, and resources for further learning. By incorporating these insights into your grooming routine, you're not only maintaining your dog's appearance but also contributing to their happiness, health, and the cherished relationship you share. Enjoy the grooming process as an opportunity to show your love and care for your loyal companion, fostering a beautiful, lifelong connection.

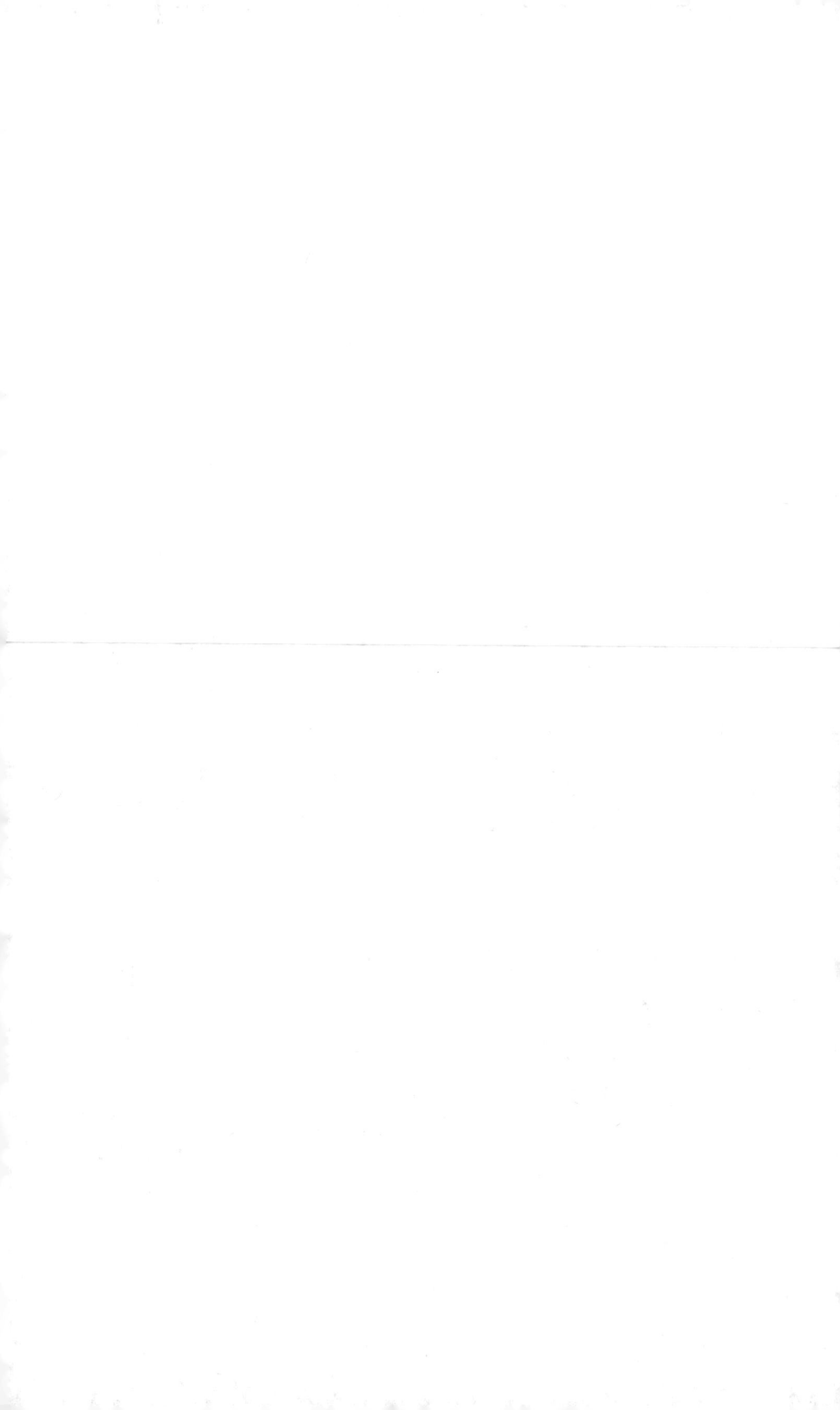

www.ingramcontent.com/pod-product-compliance
Lightning Source LLC
Chambersburg PA
CBHW070728260726
48660CB00007B/2769